52
Weeks

TO

BETTER
MENTAL
HEALTH

chartwell
books

A GUIDED WORKBOOK FOR
SELF-EXPLORATION & GROWTH

52
Weeks

BETTER
MENTAL
HEALTH

TINA B. TESSINA, PH.D., L.M.F.T.

chartwell
books

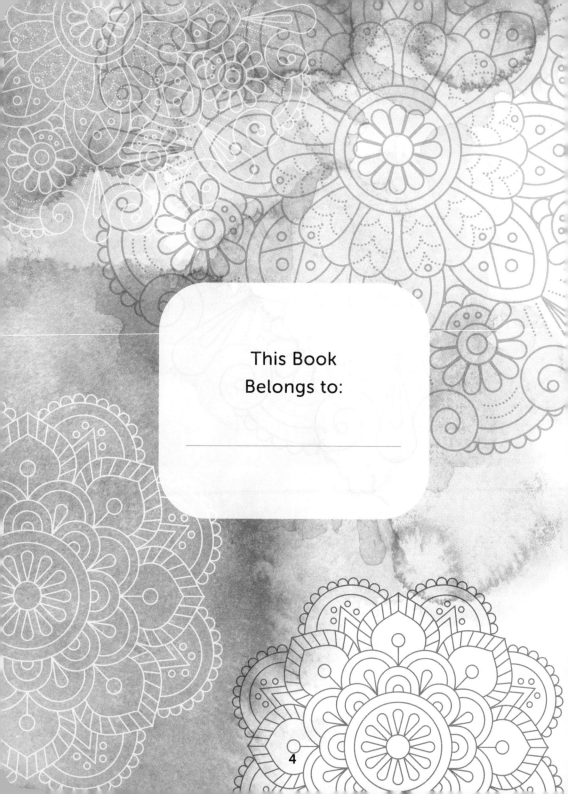

This Book
Belongs to:

_____

Introduction

If you picked up this book because you'd like to feel calmer, happier, and more comfortable in your life and in your relationships, then you came to the right place. The easy exercises in these pages will help you improve your attitude, your sense of well-being, and your satisfaction with your life.

I have been a licensed psychotherapist in private practice for more than forty years. I've helped people feel better and happier by supporting them through the difficult stages of their lives; showing them how to improve their relationships and connections with partners, family, and friends; and teaching them how to tame their out-of-control emotions and learn emotional self-management. The exercises and writing prompts in this book are similar to the homework I give my clients each week to help them understand themselves and each other. Using these tools as a basis for your personal exploration will guide you along your journey of self-discovery and healing.

Additionally, I'll help you develop your own "life hacks" or mental tricks that can help your daily routines go smoother, help you be more productive, and help you feel more balanced between working/producing and playing/relaxing. You'll find out how to:

* motivate yourself (and by extension, others);

* create and maintain happier relationships;

* have more balance between work and restorative relaxation;

* feel more in charge and organized in managing your time;

* deal with problematic people;

* manage difficult feelings, like anger, grief, and anxiety; and

* set and maintain appropriate goals for your unique set of skills and attributes.

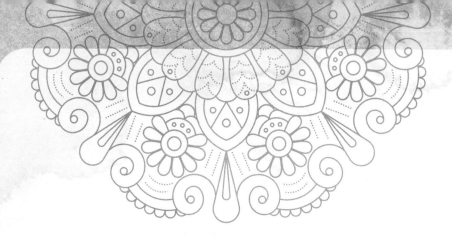

To do all these things requires you to become familiar with your feelings and thoughts. Most of us spend more time blocking out our feelings and thoughts than we do honoring them, but discovering who you really are is a powerful way to create change. During the year covered in this book, you will learn to become aware of your hidden feelings and thoughts, to become familiar with them, and to learn to manage them more easily. As you learn this, you'll find you're no longer blindsided by unexpected emotions or affected by unbidden thoughts that can cause anxiety, depression, and/or inappropriate or angry outbursts.

At its most basic, your mental health is your relationship with yourself, your thoughts, and your emotions. Improve those things, which is easier than you might think, and you'll improve all your other relationships as well.

Becoming Familiar with Hidden Thoughts

Our conscious thoughts use only a small portion of our brains. Much of the brain is occupied by things we don't think about: breathing, blood circulation and pressure, automatic reflexes, walking, vision, taste, hearing, talking, and other bodily functions we tend to take for granted. Our bodies just seem to work without our conscious interference. For example, your native language may seem to be there when you need it, but if you've ever learned a foreign language as an adult, you can feel how much brain power goes into language learning.

Another large part of the brain is devoted to feelings, memories, dreams, fantasies, spirituality, and emotional energy. The term I prefer for this part of our minds is the subconscious. All our memories, reactions, feelings, and a lot of thinking goes on just below our awareness, but it can have profound effects on who we feel we are, how we interact with others, and even on autonomic body functions like blood pressure and heartbeat. If you've ever struggled with your blood pressure being abnormally high just because you're at the doctor's office (known as "white coat syndrome") or felt your heart race because you're watching an exciting game or seeing someone you have strong feelings for, you know thoughts and feelings can affect you physically. Subconscious thoughts can also create unpleasant emotional reactions like anxiety attacks, and suppressed grieving is often behind depression.

Our goal in this little book is to help you become familiar with your hidden thoughts and feelings so you can manage them and resolve them—and no longer be at the mercy of them.

—Tina B. Tessina, PH.D., L.M.F.T.

How to Use This Workbook

Regularly writing down thoughts, feelings, and goals can ultimately help reduce stress, increase focus, ease anxiety, improve positivity, and just make life work better overall. Following guided writing prompts takes the personal discovery one step further by helping you attune to your mental and emotional needs in ways that can help you increase your total well-being. Writing is one of the best ways to examine and sort out your feelings. It can help you put your life into perspective and figure out what's important to you and where you want to go next.

52 Weeks to Better Mental Health offers focused self-exploration exercises for every week of the year, so you can start your fifty-two weeks at any point, on any day, in any season, and work through the exercises until you've completed a year. Although it should take a year to do all the exercises, you'll start to notice a difference very quickly because you'll find prompts designed to help you look at yourself and your life from a new perspective, which will have a noticeable effect in a short time. The fifty-two weeks are divided into nine sections, each with several weeks of prompts to help you progress through mastery of the topic. Some sections are shorter than others, but they are organized in the manner that most of my clients progress through while improving their mental health.

You'll also find helpful explanations, encouraging quotes, and affirmations every week. Further, every other week offers additional check-ins for self-reflection on progress and goal setting. As you continue your journey, you'll notice that you're more comfortable with your inner thoughts and feelings—and happier with who you are.

This workbook can also help you:

Reduce stress
It shows you how to observe your mental process without obsessing and worrying fruitlessly.

Order your thinking
When you write things down in an orderly fashion, you can prioritize them.

Organize
It shows you how to think logically about whatever you want to do.

Focus
Getting your thoughts in an orderly form helps you track them and figure out what you want to know.

Improve your well-being
Calming your racing thoughts reduces stress, expresses pent-up emotions, and helps you think clearly about them and decide what you want to do.

Make time for you
Writing is like a love letter to yourself, and it makes it clear that you care about you, which is a boost to healthy self-esteem.

Make this the workbook for creating the life you want. Explore yourself—and improve your mental outlook—through one year of self-reflective writing prompts. There's no way to make a mistake here, and the only one who'll see your musings will be you. Let's begin.

1

Mental Health & Self-Awareness

We all have leftovers from the past: old problems, hurts, and memories that can trouble us on an ongoing basis. Everyone also has an "internal dialog" that often includes hurtful words and beliefs from our pasts that we unconsciously retained because they were painful or concerning. These harsh phrases tend to run on a loop just below our awareness. Whether the mental leftovers come from childhood, a destructive relationship, or a negative work environment, you don't have to live with them. You can learn to replace them with internal dialog that is encouraging rather than discouraging, motivating rather than destructive, and healing rather than upsetting. To do that, you need to become aware of the hidden, inner dialog you have with yourself, and these next few weeks are designed to help you do that.

Meet Yourself

Use the "selfie" option on your phone's camera or a mirror to take a look at yourself. Say "hello" and smile. What are your thoughts about you when you see yourself?

_____

_____

_____

_____

_____

_____

_____

_____

If the thoughts are critical, can you turn them around to be more positive?

_____

_____

_____

_____

_____

_____

_____

> *"What lies behind us and what lies ahead of us are tiny matters compared to what lives within us."* —HENRY DAVID THOREAU

How can you be a better friend to yourself?

_____

_____

_____

_____

_____

_____

Write some positive things you can say to yourself. Set a reminder on your phone to remind you to say something nice to yourself every hour. If you do this consistently for this week, and then keep it going on a timeline that suits you, you'll develop a healthy habit that will enhance your well-being.

_____

_____

_____

_____

_____

Choose a Name

**I am often surprised by the nasty names
my clients call themselves, like "stupid" or "worthless."
Here's a chance to change that.**

Choose a name for your Inner Self: It could be a childhood nickname, your own name with "Little" in front of it, or something someone once called you that made you feel special. Be careful not to choose a name that doesn't feel good to you. Repeat the name often, until it becomes second nature. My name for myself is "Punkin" because a dear friend calls me that. What is yours?

I call my Inner Self: _____

What do you think of when you call yourself by this name?

_____

_____

_____

_____

_____

Write a short letter or note to yourself using your chosen name and describing the friendship you would like to have with yourself.

A name represents identity, a deep feeling and holds tremendous significance to its owner." —RACHEL INGBER

How does it feel to give yourself an affectionate name?

_____

_____

_____

_____

_____

_____

_____

Write yourself a brief note every day, either here or on sticky notes, using your affectionate nickname. For example, "Dear Punkin: Have fun today."

_____

_____

_____

_____

_____

_____

_____

_____

_____

_____

Reflections

What surprised you about yourself these past two weeks?

_____

_____

_____

_____

_____

Did you learn something new?

_____

_____

_____

_____

_____

Can you put your new awareness into action?

_____

_____

_____

_____

_____

Make Friends with Yourself

Think of someone in your life, past or present, for whom you care. How would you greet them?

_____

_____

_____

_____

_____

_____

_____

_____

_____

Greet your new friend, your Inner Self, by your affectionate nickname in the same way. Write that here.

_____

_____

_____

Using your imagination, take your Inner Self on a virtual tour of your living space. Point out what you love about your space and write it here.

_____

_____

_____

_____

_____

_____

_____

_____

Choose a place for your new friend to live in your space and describe it here.

_____

_____

_____

_____

_____

_____

_____

_____

_____

_____

_____

"Oh the comfort... of feeling safe with a person, having neither to weigh thoughts, nor measure words, but pouring them all out, just as they are, chaff and grain together; knowing that a faithful hand will take and sift them...and with the breath of kindness blow the rest away."

—DINAH MARIA CRAIK

Using your affectionate nickname, welcome your new friend to your space. For example, "Dear Punkin: You live here now, with me. You have a special place to be, and you're safe here."

_____

_____

_____

_____

_____

_____

_____

Develop Your Friendship

Begin a habit of writing to your new inner friend every day.

_____

_____

_____

_____

_____

_____

_____

_____

_____

_____

_____

_____

_____

_____

_____

_____

_____

_____

_____

_____

Take your new inner friend on a walk and write about it here.

_____

_____

_____

_____

_____

_____

_____

_____

Did things look different when you had your friend along?

_____

_____

_____

_____

_____

_____

_____

_____

_____

_____

*"Of all possessions a friend
is the most precious."*

—HERODOTUS

What did you notice especially?

_____

_____

_____

_____

_____

_____

What is your inner friend saying to you?

_____

_____

_____

_____

_____

_____

_____

Reflections

What surprised you about yourself these past two weeks?

_____
_____
_____
_____
_____

Did you learn something new?

_____
_____
_____
_____
_____

Can you put your new awareness into action?

_____
_____
_____
_____
_____

2

Managing Conflicting Thoughts

When you're agitated by a lot of ideas swirling around in your head, such as what others want you to do, what you want to do, and all the choices you have, writing things down can help you sort out all the facts, eliminate the bad ideas, and reach a conclusion that you can feel confident about. After writing and analyzing your thoughts, you'll know your solution is the right one for you. If you make your decision without the benefit of this process of self-awareness, you may not feel certain that your decision is truly your own. And if people you respect or care for have voiced an opinion about the decision, consciously honoring your own perspective is all the more important.

Listen to Yourself

Most of us ask other people what they think of events, feelings, and problems in our lives, but we often forget to ask ourselves what we think.

Identify something you need to decide, and ask your own opinion: What do *you* think about whatever is happening in your life?

_____

_____

_____

_____

_____

_____

Now write the pros and cons about your decision here.

_____

_____

_____

_____

_____

_____

Review your pros and cons: What do you think is most important?

_____

_____

_____

_____

What worries you? What do you feel good about?

_____

_____

_____

_____

What is your best option?

_____

_____

_____

_____

_____

"Courage is what it takes to stand up and speak; courage is also what it takes to sit down and listen." —WINSTON CHURCHILL

Give Yourself Advice

If you were speaking to a friend (which you are), how would you advise them about their current choices? Give the same sort of advice to yourself.

_____

_____

_____

_____

How can you encourage yourself?

_____

_____

_____

_____

Motivation comes from celebration and appreciation. Turn the page and work through the week. Then make a list of what you've gotten done this week and congratulate yourself for each item on the list.

_____

_____

_____

MORNING EXERCISE

Every morning this week, write down what your focus for the day will be and what you'd like to accomplish.

Day #1 Focus: _____

Today I will: _____
_____
_____
_____

Day #2 Focus: _____

Today I will: _____
_____
_____
_____

Day #3 Focus: _____

Today I will: _____
_____
_____
_____

Day #4 Focus: _____

Today I will: _____
_____
_____
_____

Day #5 Focus: _____

Today I will: _____
_____
_____
_____

Day #6 Focus: _____

Today I will: _____
_____
_____
_____

Day #7 Focus: _____

Today I will: _____
_____
_____
_____

Additional notes: _____
_____
_____
_____

EVENING EXERCISE

Review your day, celebrate what you accomplished (even getting out of bed), and consider what you'd do differently.

Day #1 Today I accomplished:

_____
_____
_____

What I could differently: _____
_____
_____

Day #2 Today I accomplished:

_____
_____
_____

What I could differently: _____
_____
_____

Day #3 Today I accomplished:

_____
_____
_____

What I could differently: _____
_____
_____

Day #4 Today I accomplished:

_____
_____
_____

What I could differently: _____
_____
_____

Day #5 Today I accomplished:

_____
_____
_____

What I could differently: _____
_____
_____

Day #6 Today I accomplished:

_____
_____
_____

What I could differently: _____
_____
_____

Day #7 Today I accomplished:

_____
_____
_____

What I could differently: _____
_____
_____

Additional notes: _____
_____
_____
_____
_____
_____

Reflections

What surprised you about yourself these past two weeks?

_____

_____

_____

_____

_____

Did you learn something new?

_____

_____

_____

_____

_____

Can you put your new awareness into action?

_____

_____

_____

_____

_____

Be Kind

Consider the advice you gave yourself in the last week: Was it kind and supportive?

_____

_____

_____

_____

_____

_____

_____

How can you make it more supportive?

_____

_____

_____

_____

_____

_____

_____

> *"No act of kindness, no matter how small, is ever wasted."*
>
> —AESOP

Think of the kindest person you know. What would that person say to you?

_____

_____

_____

_____

_____

_____

What unkind thoughts are you aware of? Can you change them to be kind and supportive?

_____

_____

_____

_____

_____

_____

_____

Practice saying kind and supportive things to yourself this week. List five of them here.

1. _____
_____

2. _____
_____

3. _____
_____

4. _____
_____

5. _____
_____

3

Stress & Resistance

Knowing how to manage your stress is essential to having good mental health. A certain amount of stress from life is inevitable, but there are healthy and unhealthy ways of handling it. Better stress management improves your ability to think clearly and make good choices. Unmanaged stress has harmful effects on your physical body, such as raising blood pressure and heart rate and lowering your immune response, among other things. Resistance is an internal thought habit that creates stress; because internal stress is self-created, you can learn *not* to create it. In these next few weeks, we'll focus on eliminating internal stress and reducing the effects of external stress.

Understanding Your Stress

What creates stress in your life?

_____

_____

_____

_____

_____

_____

_____

Do you get stressed about things you haven't done or when your to-do list piles up?

_____

_____

_____

_____

_____

_____

_____

_____

Do relationships cause you stress and in what ways?

_____

_____

_____

_____

_____

_____

Do you bring work stress home with you, and how does that manifest?

_____

_____

_____

_____

_____

_____

Does worrying about what stresses you keep you from sleeping well?

_____

_____

_____

_____

_____

_____

Reflections

What surprised you about yourself these past two weeks?

_____

_____

_____

_____

_____

Did you learn something new?

_____

_____

_____

_____

Can you put your new awareness into action?

_____

_____

_____

_____

Self-Talk to Handle Stress

If a friend of yours were stressed about the same things as you, what would you say to that friend?

_____

_____

_____

_____

_____

_____

_____

Try saying the same things to yourself. Does it calm you down?

_____

_____

_____

_____

_____

_____

_____

> *"There is only one corner of the universe you can be certain of improving, and that's your own self."* —ALDOUS HUXLEY

Look at your list of what creates stress for you, from page 35, and order it from most to least stressful.

_____

_____

_____

_____

_____

_____

_____

_____

Consider the most stressful thing on your list. Is it happening now, in the past, or in the future? Now mark each item with Past, Now, or Future.

If your most stressful thing is happening now, consider what you may do to solve the problem. Is there anything you can do right now, help you can get, online research, or a friend to ask for advice?

"I have great respect for the past. If you don't know where you've come from, you don't know where you're going." —MAYA ANGELOU

Stress & Expectations

If you came up with a possible solution to something on your list of stressful things, put it into action. If not, consider what you'll do if the worst possible thing happens.

_____

_____

_____

_____

_____

_____

What if the best possible outcome happens?

_____

_____

_____

_____

_____

_____

Does thinking of the outcome suggest any possible solutions?

_____
_____
_____
_____
_____
_____
_____
_____
_____

Find something you can do, no matter how small (like looking up information, asking for help, or trying something you're not sure will work). Write it here, then do it.

_____
_____
_____
_____
_____
_____
_____
_____
_____

Once you've done *anything* about the problem, celebrate what you've done, even if it didn't fix everything. How did you celebrate?

_____

_____

_____

_____

_____

_____

_____

_____

_____

_____

"If you accept the expectations of others, especially negative ones, then you never will change the outcome." —MICHAEL JORDAN

Reflections

What surprised you about yourself these past two weeks?

_____

_____

_____

_____

_____

Did you learn something new?

_____

_____

_____

_____

_____

Can you put your new awareness into action?

_____

_____

_____

_____

_____

Stress & Confronting Problems

Write down: "I'm stressed about _____

_____

_____,

so I'm going to tackle it. It's less stressful to do what's necessary than to worry about it."

Say it out loud, whisper it, or mumble it under your breath to yourself, then write it again.

_____

_____

_____

_____

"The greatest weapon against stress is our ability to choose one thought over another." —WILLIAM JAMES

When you say it or write it, do you hear a response in your mind? (e.g., "It's too hard" or "You can't make me!" or "I don't want to" or "I might mess it up!") What you hear is your resistance. Resistance has a place (more about that later), but not when you're resisting something you want or need to get done. Write down all your resistance.

What do you want to say to your resistance? (Strive to be as positive as you can.)

_____

_____

_____

_____

_____

_____

_____

_____

_____

_____

"You will find peace not by trying to escape your problems, but by confronting them courageously. You will find peace not in denial, but in victory." —J. DONALD WALTERS

Stress & Self-Soothing

What would your parents say or do to comfort you when you were sick or hurt as a child?

_____

_____

_____

_____

_____

_____

_____

How did that make you feel?

_____

_____

_____

_____

_____

_____

_____

_____

"Expect trouble as an inevitable part of life and repeat to yourself the most comforting words of all: 'This, too, shall pass.'" —ANN LANDERS

Was there anything you wanted to be told or have done for you that you didn't get?

_____

_____

_____

_____

_____

_____

_____

Learning from those examples, list five ways you can comfort yourself.

1. _____
2. _____
3. _____
4. _____
5. _____

How can you create a habit of comforting yourself when you need it?

_____

_____

_____

_____

_____

_____

_____

_____

_____

_____

"Believe in yourself! Have faith in your abilities! Without a humble but reasonable confidence in your own powers you cannot be successful or happy."

—NORMAN VINCENT PEALE

Reflections

What surprised you about yourself these past two weeks?

_____

_____

_____

_____

Did you learn something new?

_____

_____

_____

_____

Can you put your new awareness into action?

_____

_____

_____

_____

Chronic Fixes for Chronic Problems

What problems keep occurring in your life?

_____

_____

_____

_____

_____

_____

_____

_____

What have you tried that seemed to work for each problem?

_____

_____

_____

_____

_____

_____

_____

_____

_____

What new things have you tried to resolve each problem?

_____

_____

_____

_____

_____

_____

_____

_____

_____

_____

Get help from your Inner Self: What does that part of you need to resolve the problems?

_____

_____

_____

_____

_____

_____

_____

_____

_____

When a problem recurs, have you tried using what worked before to solve it?

_____

_____

_____

_____

_____

_____

_____

_____

_____

_____

_____

_____

"Don't continually look for new solutions. First, use the ones that worked before."

—TINA B. TESSINA

Confronting Resistance

Resistance can be your friend—when you need to stand up for yourself to others, or to control your problematic impulses—but when it's just stubbornness getting in your way, you need to learn to handle it.

How did you do with your resistance?

_____

_____

_____

_____

_____

Explain to yourself why what you want to do is worth doing.

_____

_____

_____

_____

_____

Explain the rewards you'll get from doing what you're resisting.

_____

_____

_____

_____

_____

_____

_____

_____

_____

Ask your Inner Self to work with you, and promise (sincerely) that you will work with your Inner Self and be a team. Make an agreement with yourself and write it here.

_____

_____

_____

_____

_____

_____

_____

_____

_____

_____

"What is needed, rather than running away or controlling or suppressing or any other resistance, is understanding fear; that means watch it, learn about it, come directly into contact with it. We are to learn about fear, not how to escape from it."

—JIDDU KRISHNAMURTI

How does your agreement feel to both your inner and outer self?

Reflections

What surprised you about yourself these past two weeks?

_____

_____

_____

_____

_____

Did you learn something new?

_____

_____

_____

_____

_____

Can you put your new awareness into action?

_____

_____

_____

_____

_____

Rethinking

If you have very strong resistance to doing something, consider there may be a good reason. (For example, your body or your Inner Self is trying to tell you your solution is too stressful, or you're trying to do too much in too short a time.) What is your resistance about?

_____

_____

_____

_____

_____

_____

Are you sure doing it will be valuable to you?

_____

_____

_____

_____

_____

_____

Are you doing it because you want to, or because you think others expect it of you?

_____

_____

_____

_____

_____

_____

_____

_____

Are you trying to please someone rather than meet a goal?

_____

_____

_____

_____

_____

_____

_____

_____

_____

Consider what doing the thing you're resisting will accomplish for you. Is it worthwhile?

_____

_____

_____

_____

_____

_____

_____

_____

_____

_____

"We should not give up and we should not allow the problem to defeat us."

—A. P. J. ABDUL KALAM

4

Building Confidence & Trust

A major benefit of being connected to yourself and in charge of your decisions is the big boost you get in self-confidence. Self-confidence, or the ability to trust yourself, helps you navigate your life successfully and approach new situations calmly and competently. Being a good friend to yourself leads to trusting yourself, and trusting yourself builds your confidence. These next few weeks will guide you in building your confidence and trust.

Build Confidence

How well do you trust yourself?

_____

_____

_____

_____

_____

_____

_____

Where and how do you let yourself down?

_____

_____

_____

_____

_____

_____

_____

How well do you keep your promises to others?

_____

_____

_____

_____

_____

Do you keep promises you make to yourself?

_____

_____

_____

_____

_____

_____

How does your trustworthiness with yourself impact your
trustworthiness with others?

_____

_____

_____

_____

_____

_____

Reflections

What surprised you about yourself these past two weeks?

_____

_____

_____

_____

Did you learn something new?

_____

_____

_____

_____

Can you put your new awareness into action?

_____

_____

_____

_____

Your History of Trust

Who have you trusted in the past?

_____

_____

_____

_____

_____

_____

_____

_____

_____

Who let you down?

_____

_____

_____

_____

_____

_____

_____

_____

_____

_____

How did that feel?

_____

_____

_____

_____

_____

_____

_____

"Trust is the glue of life. It's the most essential ingredient in effective communication. It's the foundational principle that holds all relationships."

—STEPHEN COVEY

Who turned out to be reliable?

_____

_____

_____

_____

_____

_____

How can you be more like the trustworthy people in your past?

_____

_____

_____

_____

_____

_____

_____

_____

Knowing Who to Trust

What were the characteristics of trustworthy people in your past?

_____

_____

_____

_____

_____

_____

_____

_____

What were the personality traits and habits of the untrustworthy people?

_____

_____

_____

_____

_____

_____

_____

_____

Are the people you know today trustworthy?

How trustworthy are you to your friends and family?

How trustworthy are you to yourself?

"He who does not trust enough will not be trusted."

—LAOZI (LAO TZU)

Reflections

What surprised you about yourself these past two weeks?

_____

_____

_____

_____

_____

Did you learn something new?

_____

_____

_____

_____

Can you put your new awareness into action?

_____

_____

_____

_____

Changing How You Trust

Thinking about the people you can trust, what do they say to you?

_____

_____

_____

_____

_____

_____

_____

_____

What do the trustworthy people do?

_____

_____

_____

_____

_____

_____

_____

Do their words fit their actions?

_____
_____
_____
_____
_____
_____
_____
_____
_____
_____
_____
_____
_____

"What we learn only through
the ears makes less impression
upon our minds than what is
presented to the trustworthy eye."

—HORACE

Using them as a model, what should you look for to trust someone?

_____

_____

_____

_____

_____

_____

_____

_____

True trust builds slowly. How does it develop between you and others?

_____

_____

_____

_____

_____

_____

_____

_____

_____

Use Your Judgment

There's a difference between being judgmental and using judgment. You don't have to say critical things about people, but you do need to pay attention to whether they're trustworthy and use your judgment.

Using what you've learned in week 19 about trustworthy people, what should your criteria be for deciding if someone is trustworthy?

_____

_____

_____

_____

_____

_____

_____

_____

_____

_____

_____

_____

You don't have to trust everyone in your life. Of the people you know, who is trustworthy and who is not?

_____

_____

_____

_____

If you can trust yourself, it's not so important whether others are trustworthy. Why is this true?

_____

_____

_____

_____

_____

_____

When you're getting to know a new person, how do you begin to tell if they're trustworthy?

_____

_____

_____

_____

_____

_____

What have you observed about the people in your life and whether you can trust them?

_____

_____

_____

_____

_____

_____

_____

_____

_____

_____

_____

"Depend upon yourself. Make your judgment trustworthy by trusting it. You can develop good judgment as you do the muscles of your body—by judicious, daily exercise." —GRANTLAND RICE

Reflections

What surprised you about yourself these past two weeks?

_____

_____

_____

_____

_____

Did you learn something new?

_____

_____

_____

_____

_____

Can you put your new awareness into action?

_____

_____

_____

_____

_____

Build Your Confidence

How can you be a good friend to yourself?

_____
_____
_____
_____
_____
_____
_____
_____
_____

Do you reassure and support yourself?

_____
_____
_____
_____
_____
_____
_____
_____
_____

Are you checking in with yourself every day?

_____

_____

_____

_____

_____

_____

_____

_____

Do you listen carefully to yourself and take what you hear seriously?

_____

_____

_____

_____

_____

_____

_____

_____

_____

_____

How can you be more supportive and reassuring to yourself?

_____

_____

_____

_____

_____

_____

_____

_____

_____

_____

_____

"Kindness begins with the understanding that we all struggle."

—CHARLES GLASSMAN

5

Getting in Charge of Your Life

It sometimes seems easy to drift along and let life happen, but at the end of the drifting, you can feel dissatisfied and somewhat mystified with the result. These next few weeks will help you get in charge of what you're doing each day and for the future.

Making Plans

Imagine the life you'd like to have a few years from now and write about it here.

_____

_____

_____

_____

_____

_____

_____

_____

What steps are required to accomplish your plan or goal?

_____

_____

_____

_____

_____

_____

_____

_____

Review the steps to make sure they are small enough to accomplish; if not, break them down smaller.

Choose a step and do it. How did it feel?

How can you celebrate your accomplishment, no matter how small it is?

Reflections

What surprised you about yourself these past two weeks?

_____
_____
_____
_____
_____

Did you learn something new?

_____
_____
_____
_____

Can you put your new awareness into action?

_____
_____
_____
_____

Creating Success

How did you do at making plans and then taking and celebrating your steps?

_____

_____

_____

_____

_____

_____

_____

_____

What could you do differently to improve your success?

_____

_____

_____

_____

_____

_____

_____

_____

Did you break down your goal into steps—and do the steps need to be smaller? For example, if your goal is to get a degree, the first step could be "search for schools." Each step should feel easy as the previous ones are completed.

_____

_____

_____

_____

_____

_____

_____

_____

Did you choose a step and do it? If not, choose one. If you did, choose the next step. Write it here.

_____

_____

_____

_____

_____

_____

_____

_____

_____

If a step is too hard, break it down into smaller actions until it feels easy. Write them here.

"Success always demands greater effort."

—WINSTON CHURCHILL

Celebration = Motivation

What kind of simple celebrations work for you?

_____

_____

_____

_____

_____

_____

_____

_____

What was your favorite celebration in childhood (e.g., a cookie, a balloon, time spent with a parent/siblings/friends)?

_____

_____

_____

_____

_____

_____

_____

Can you create a similar but simple celebration that makes your child-self happy? (Perhaps some balloon or gold star stickers you could put next to the completed steps of your plan? Or call a sibling or friend when you finish a step?)

When you celebrate a completed step, do you notice a boost in your spirit or energy for the next one?

What have you completed and celebrated?

_____
_____
_____
_____
_____
_____
_____
_____
_____
_____
_____
_____
_____

"Celebration +
Appreciation =
Motivation."

—TINA B. TESSINA

Reflections

What surprised you about yourself these past two weeks?

_____

_____

_____

_____

Did you learn something new?

_____

_____

_____

_____

Can you put your new awareness into action?

_____

_____

_____

_____

6

Other People & You

Good mental health involves not only yourself but other people too. Your relationships with others are based on your relationship with yourself. What other people do is not your fault or your responsibility. Your responsibility lies in how you respond to what others say and do. These next few weeks will help you navigate that.

Circles of Friends

We all have various circles of friends, from casual acquaintances to deep friendships. Even family members vary in their closeness to us. If you understand this, you'll be more careful in trusting.

Think of your friends forming a series of concentric circles. The closest ones to you, the most trustworthy, are few. There are more people in the circles as they expand. Who is in your **innermost circle**? (Don't forget to include yourself.)

_____

_____

_____

_____

The **second circle** is good friends, but not the closest ones. Who is in the second circle?

_____

_____

_____

_____

_____

The **third circle** is casual friends, friends of friends, etc. Who are they?

_____

_____

_____

_____

_____

_____

The **fourth circle** is circumstantial friends, like the person you may frequently have lunch with at work, but if you changed jobs you wouldn't see them again. Who are they?

_____

_____

_____

_____

_____

Do you think your friends have you in their same circles? Why or why not?

_____

_____

_____

_____

_____

_____

Managing Friendships

People can move in and out of your circles of friendship as circumstances, which you may have no control over, change.

As your life has progressed, who has grown closer to you?

_____

_____

_____

_____

_____

_____

_____

Who has grown farther apart?

_____

_____

_____

_____

_____

Who do you know that you would like to be closer to?

_____

_____

_____

_____

_____

_____

_____

_____

_____

What would make you want to be closer to someone?

_____

_____

_____

_____

_____

_____

_____

_____

_____

_____

_____

What can you do to invite someone closer?

"Everyone thinks of changing the world, but no one thinks of changing himself."

—LEO TOLSTOY

Reflections

What surprised you about yourself these past two weeks?

_____
_____
_____
_____
_____

Did you learn something new?

_____
_____
_____
_____

Can you put your new awareness into action?

_____
_____
_____
_____
_____

How Friends Treat You

Of the people close to you, who treats you as you want to be treated?

_____

_____

_____

_____

_____

_____

Is there anyone who treats you differently now than they did before? What could be the reason for that?

_____

_____

_____

_____

_____

_____

_____

Considering your circles of friendship, who has moved closer? Put them in their new positions in your circles.

_____

_____

_____

_____

_____

_____

_____

_____

_____

Who has moved farther away in your circles? Put them in their new positions.

_____

_____

_____

_____

_____

_____

_____

_____

_____

> *"We are not the same persons this year as last; nor are those we love. It is a happy chance if we, changing, continue to love a changed person."*
>
> —W. SOMERSET MAUGHAM

On which people do you want to place your positive attention? Why is this so?

_____

_____

_____

_____

_____

_____

_____

_____

_____

_____

_____

Getting What You Want from Friendship

What do you want from your friends? Fun? Support? Challenges? Loyalty?

_____

_____

_____

_____

_____

_____

_____

How are you giving those things to yourself?

_____

_____

_____

_____

_____

_____

_____

Is there something you want from a particular person?

"Change will not come if we wait for some other person or some other time. We are the ones we've been waiting for. We are the change that we seek."

—BARACK OBAMA

How can you give that to yourself?

_____

_____

_____

_____

_____

_____

_____

When you give yourself what you want, do your friendships
seem different?

_____

_____

_____

_____

_____

_____

_____

_____

_____

_____

Reflections

What surprised you about yourself these past two weeks?

_____

_____

_____

_____

Did you learn something new?

_____

_____

_____

_____

Can you put your new awareness into action?

_____

_____

_____

_____

Handling Grief & Loss

Loving friends, family, and pets means we will lose some of them sooner or later. Some will just move out of your circles, perhaps to become more long-distance friendships; some you will lose touch with; and some will pass away. Relationships also ebb and flow. Even if a relationship is flawed, we must grieve the loss. It's the nature of life, and the older you get, the more grief and loss you will experience. Learning to move through the grief process is an essential life skill.

What friends, loved ones, or pets have you lost?

_____

_____

_____

How do you remember them?

_____

_____

_____

_____

_____

_____

Honoring your grief is honoring your love for the lost one. How do you honor your grief?

_____

_____

_____

_____

_____

_____

_____

_____

Expressing your grief is also honoring your lost ones. How can you express your grief?

_____

_____

_____

_____

_____

_____

_____

_____

Tell someone you lost whatever you want to tell them. Write it here.

_____

_____

_____

_____

_____

_____

_____

_____

_____

_____

"Any natural, normal human being, when faced with any kind of loss, will go from shock all the way through acceptance."

—ELISABETH KÜBLER-ROSS

Making New Friends

The only friendship you will have birth to death is the one with yourself. Because people change, circumstances change, and life and love involve loss and grief, learning to make new friends is essential.

To make new friends with whom you have something in common, do things regularly that involve others. This makes developing friendships easier. What new things can you do that involve other people with similar interests?

_____

_____

_____

_____

_____

_____

_____

_____

_____

_____

_____

_____

_____

When you find someone you think is particularly pleasant, spend a little time talking with them during or after your activity. If the conversation goes well, you can offer to meet before or after the session for coffee. Whom have you met that you want to ask for coffee?

_____

_____

_____

_____

While you're making new friends, don't forget the people you already know. Is there a favorite family member or an acquaintance you'd like to see more often? Whom do you already know that you'd like to call and suggest going for a walk or to lunch?

_____

_____

_____

_____

If you are turned down, don't get discouraged. Move on to other people. Who else would you like to ask?

_____

_____

_____

_____

Rely on your internal friendship to guide you in making new friends. What does your Inner Self say to do?

_____

_____

_____

_____

_____

_____

_____

_____

_____

"new friends can often have a better time together than old friends."

—F. SCOTT FITZGERALD

Reflections

What surprised you about yourself these past two weeks?

_____
_____
_____
_____
_____

Did you learn something new?

_____
_____
_____
_____
_____

Can you put your new awareness into action?

_____
_____
_____
_____
_____

Being Your Own Boss

Whether you work for an external boss or not, you will benefit from consciously being your own boss.

Who do you feel is in charge of your thoughts, feelings, and actions?

_____

_____

_____

_____

_____

_____

Do you ever feel out of control of your thoughts or feelings?

_____

_____

_____

_____

_____

_____

You have the power to be your own boss. How can you take charge and be more in control of yourself?

_____

_____

_____

_____

_____

_____

_____

_____

_____

_____

_____

_____

_____

_____

_____

"The greatest gift of leadership is a boss who wants you to be successful."

—JON TAFFER

What's the difference between a boss (on the job) who motivates you and one who discourages you?

_____

_____

_____

_____

_____

_____

_____

_____

_____

What would it be like to be a good boss to yourself?

_____

_____

_____

_____

_____

_____

_____

_____

_____

Motivation

As noted in Week 24, motivation comes from celebration and appreciation. This means you have the power to increase your motivation by celebrating and appreciating your accomplishments. Even when no one else is being appreciative, you can appreciate yourself.

As your own boss, how can you celebrate and appreciate what you do?

_____

_____

_____

_____

_____

_____

_____

_____

_____

_____

_____

_____

What kinds of celebrations are simple, easy, and effective for you?

_____

_____

_____

_____

What kinds of daily celebrations could you do to celebrate all
the little or big things you've accomplished?

_____

_____

_____

_____

_____

"Trust yourself. Create the kind of
self that you will be happy to live
with all your life. Make the most of
yourself by fanning the tiny, inner
sparks of possibility into flames of
achievement." —GOLDA MEIR

Morning Exercise: Every morning this week, from the perspective of your own boss, write down what your focus for the day will be and what you'd like to accomplish today.

_____

_____

_____

_____

_____

_____

_____

_____

_____

Evening Exercise: From the perspective of your own boss, review each day, celebrate what you accomplished (even getting out of bed), and consider what you would like to do differently. Encourage yourself to make the change.

_____

_____

_____

_____

_____

_____

_____

_____

_____

Reflections

What surprised you about yourself these past two weeks?

_____

_____

_____

_____

_____

Did you learn something new?

_____

_____

_____

_____

_____

Can you put your new awareness into action?

_____

_____

_____

_____

_____

7

Your Past & Mental Health

Past experience has a profound and lasting effect on your mental health. Some of the effects are beneficial; some are harmful. The effects don't have to be lasting. The next few weeks will help you sort through your past and its influences and help you choose what you want to change.

Understanding Your Past

How do you think your past influences your present actions?

_____

_____

_____

_____

_____

_____

_____

_____

Do any of your present fears come from your past?

_____

_____

_____

_____

_____

_____

What current choices come from your past influences?

_____

_____

_____

_____

_____

How do your past relationships with family, friends, and partners affect your life today?

_____

_____

_____

_____

_____

Write a letter to yourself about your past.

_____

_____

_____

_____

_____

_____

_____

_____

_____

Patterns from Your Past: Building Blocks

Imagine your mother (or mother figure) from your childhood. What were her personality characteristics (e.g., shy, funny, distant, warm, powerful, maternal)?

_____

_____

_____

_____

_____

_____

Imagine your father (or father figure) from your childhood. What were his personality characteristics?

_____

_____

_____

_____

_____

Picture those traits and characteristics as a pile of building blocks in front of each parent. What blocks would you choose for yourself?

_____

_____

_____

_____

_____

_____

_____

_____

If you feel you're missing some blocks, look for them in people you knew well in childhood, such as another family member (sibling, grandparent, aunt or uncle, cousin) or role model (coach, teacher, mentor, neighbor), and add them to your chosen blocks.

_____

_____

_____

_____

_____

_____

_____

You can choose to copy character traits from any role model, without taking the whole package. What will it feel like to adopt your chosen blocks as your own?

"Some believe all that parents, tutors, and kindred believe. They take their principles by inheritance and defend them as they would their estates because they are born heirs to them."

—ALAN WATTS

Reflections

What surprised you about yourself these past two weeks?

_____

_____

_____

_____

Did you learn something new?

_____

_____

_____

_____

Can you put your new awareness into action?

_____

_____

_____

_____

Role Models

In your early life, who were your role models?

_____

_____

_____

_____

_____

_____

_____

_____

What did you learn from them then?

_____

_____

_____

_____

_____

_____

_____

_____

"Having role models and mentors who I resonate with is so important—a lot of people have so many questions and may not know where to go to get answers or may not have someone who can relate enough to even answer in the first place." —RANA EL KALIOUBY

Who are your role models now?

_____

_____

_____

_____

_____

_____

What are you learning from them now?

_____

_____

_____

_____

_____

_____

_____

_____

_____

What does your Inner Self think of each of your role models?

_____

_____

_____

_____

_____

_____

_____

_____

_____

_____

_____

Creating Your Ideal Self

Using the "building blocks" exercise from Week 34, list the building blocks for each of your role models.

_____

_____

_____

_____

_____

_____

_____

_____

_____

_____

"You must be the change you wish to see in the world." —MAHATMA GANDHI

Which of these building blocks would you choose for yourself?

Have you developed or improved on any building blocks on your own?

Compile all the building blocks from these two weeks into a portrait of your own building blocks.

_____

_____

_____

_____

_____

_____

_____

_____

_____

_____

Discuss the building blocks picture of yourself with yourself. Do you like it? Would you like to change it?

_____

_____

_____

_____

_____

_____

_____

_____

_____

_____

Reflections

What surprised you about yourself these past two weeks?

Did you learn something new?

Can you put your new awareness into action?

Reassurance

Learning how to reassure yourself will help you get through the challenging moments in life.

Think about the times someone reassured you. What did they say or do?

_____

_____

_____

_____

_____

_____

_____

_____

_____

_____

_____

_____

_____

_____

_____

_____

_____

_____

_____

It is possible to reassure yourself. Using your nickname and emulating the reassurance you most enjoyed from others, write several reassuring things you can say to yourself when you need a boost.

_____

_____

_____

_____

_____

What are the most reassuring things you could say to your Inner Self?

_____

_____

_____

_____

_____

What actions can you take to feel reassured?

_____

_____

_____

_____

_____

_____

Write a reassuring and comforting note to yourself here and then read it to yourself.

_____

_____

_____

_____

_____

_____

_____

_____

_____

_____

_____

_____

_____

_____

_____

_____

_____

"Reassurance is like a warm jacket protecting you from the frost of harsh reality. It enables you to go on."

—TINA B. TESSINA

Gratitude

What are you most grateful for in your life?

_____

_____

_____

_____

_____

_____

_____

_____

_____

Who are the people you're grateful to the most?

_____

_____

_____

_____

_____

_____

_____

How would you like to express your gratitude to them?

_____
_____
_____
_____
_____
_____
_____
_____
_____
_____

What are you most grateful to yourself for?

_____
_____
_____
_____
_____
_____
_____
_____
_____
_____
_____

How would you like to express your gratitude for yourself?

_____

_____

_____

_____

_____

_____

_____

_____

_____

_____

_____

_____

_____

"Gratitude makes sense of our past, brings peace for today, and creates a vision for tomorrow."

—MELODY BEATTIE

Reflections

What surprised you about yourself these past two weeks?

_____

_____

_____

_____

Did you learn something new?

_____

_____

_____

_____

Can you put your new awareness into action?

_____

_____

_____

_____

Keeping Promises

Who has broken promises to you?

_____

_____

_____

_____

_____

How do you feel about it?

_____

_____

_____

_____

_____

_____

_____

_____

_____

_____

What promises have you made to yourself?

_____

_____

_____

_____

_____

_____

_____

_____

_____

_____

_____

"It is easy to make promises—it is hard work to keep them."

—BORIS JOHNSON

How well have you kept your promises to yourself?

How do you feel about your ability to keep your promises to yourself?

Encouraging Your Inner Self

What do other people say that encourages you?

_____

_____

_____

_____

_____

_____

_____

What do people say that could discourage you?

_____

_____

_____

_____

_____

_____

_____

_____

_____

What do you say to encourage other people?

_____

_____

_____

_____

_____

_____

What do you say to encourage yourself?

_____

_____

_____

_____

_____

_____

_____

"Correction does much, but encouragement does more."

—JOHANN WOLFGANG VON GOETHE

How can you create a habit of encouraging yourself every day?

Reflections

What surprised you about yourself these past two weeks?

_____

_____

_____

_____

Did you learn something new?

_____

_____

_____

_____

Can you put your new awareness into action?

_____

_____

_____

_____

Sleep Well

Do you feel you sleep well enough?

_____

_____

_____

_____

If not, have you asked your Inner Self what would help?

_____

_____

_____

_____

_____

"A ruffled mind makes a restless pillow." —CHARLOTTE BRONTË

A routine before bed can help your brain prepare for sleep.
What kind of before-bed routine do you have?

Try doing exactly the same routine every night before bed for a
couple of days. What is the result?

What do you need to do to create a healthy before-bed routine that will help you sleep better?

_____

_____

_____

_____

_____

_____

_____

_____

_____

_____

_____

_____

Mental Alarm Clock

Your Inner Self can help you go to sleep better each night and wake up at the right time in the morning. Ask your Inner Self for help sleeping and waking here:

_____

_____

_____

_____

_____

When you get into bed over the next few nights, ask your Inner Self to wake you up just before your alarm. What happens?

_____

_____

_____

_____

_____

_____

_____

_____

_____

Ask your Inner Self to wake you for a couple of nights in a row.
What happens?

_____

_____

_____

_____

_____

_____

_____

_____

_____

_____

Your Inner Self can remind you of many things if you take the
time to ask for the reminder. What reminders do you want to set?

_____

_____

_____

_____

_____

_____

_____

_____

What happened with your inner clock? Can you practice using your inner alarm more to get better at it?

_____

_____

_____

_____

_____

_____

_____

_____

_____

_____

_____

_____

"My aim is to wake up every morning a better person than when I went to bed."

—SIDNEY POITIER

Reflections

What surprised you about yourself these past two weeks?

_____

_____

_____

_____

Did you learn something new?

_____

_____

_____

_____

Can you put your new awareness into action?

_____

_____

_____

_____

Checking in with Yourself

How is your friendship with your Inner Self doing?

_____

_____

_____

_____

_____

_____

_____

_____

If you have been checking in with yourself daily, what have you discovered?

_____

_____

_____

_____

_____

_____

_____

What is your Inner Self asking you?

"Life is a journey, and it's about growing and changing and coming to terms with who and what you are and loving who and what you are."

—KELLY McGILLIS

What are your responses?

How do you feel about your connection with yourself?

8

Integrity: Being Your Authentic Self

Everyone seems to be looking for happiness, but many search in the wrong places. Temporary happiness can come from many things: getting high, accomplishing something, falling in love. But true, lasting happiness that doesn't fade comes from within you. It can't be bought or achieved by what you do. It's the connection with yourself that creates true happiness, and from there it spreads to others and bounces back to you.

The Source of Happiness

How happy do you feel?

_____

_____

_____

_____

_____

What represents happiness to you?

_____

_____

_____

_____

_____

_____

_____

Which other people make you happy?

_____

_____

_____

Can you be happy alone?

_____

_____

_____

_____

_____

_____

What can you do to make yourself happy?

_____

_____

_____

_____

_____

_____

_____

_____

_____

"Happiness is not a goal, it is a by-product of a life well lived."

—ELEANOR ROOSEVELT

Reflections

What surprised you about yourself these past two weeks?

_____

_____

_____

_____

Did you learn something new?

_____

_____

_____

_____

Can you put your new awareness into action?

_____

_____

_____

_____

Relating to Others while Supporting Yourself

When do you feel supported by other people?

_____

_____

_____

_____

_____

_____

_____

What do they do to support you?

_____

_____

_____

_____

_____

_____

_____

_____

Do they ever undermine you (intentionally or not)?

_____

_____

_____

_____

_____

_____

_____

_____

_____

"I feel more grounded and more settled than I ever have. . .as you age, you become more selective about what you listen to, devote your time to, and who you hang out with." —SHARON STONE

Do you support or undermine yourself?

How can you support yourself even when other people don't?

Balancing Your Inner & Outer Lives

In terms of work, play, time with yourself, and time with others, which of these do you think is out of balance in your life?

_____

_____

_____

_____

_____

_____

What can you do to balance them?

_____

_____

_____

_____

_____

_____

"It's all about quality of life and finding a happy balance between work and friends and family." —PHILIP GREEN

What does your Inner Self want to do?

_____

_____

_____

_____

_____

_____

_____

_____

_____

_____

_____

_____

_____

_____

What needs to change?

_____

_____

_____

_____

_____

_____

_____

_____

What is your plan to get your life into better balance?

_____

_____

_____

_____

_____

_____

_____

_____

_____

Reflections

What surprised you about yourself these past two weeks?

_____

_____

_____

_____

Did you learn something new?

_____

_____

_____

_____

Can you put your new awareness into action?

_____

_____

_____

_____

9

Fun & Joy

Good mental health is the key to happiness, and having fun improves mental health. These last weeks are focused on having fun, creating joy, and celebrating all you have done.

Remembering to Do the Healthy Things

After considering balance and supporting yourself, what things do you need to do regularly?

_____

_____

_____

_____

_____

_____

_____

What kinds of reminders (sticky notes, phone or calendar alarms) can you set up to remind yourself to do them regularly?

_____

_____

_____

_____

_____

_____

What interactions with your Inner Self feel life-affirming and encouraging to you?

_____

_____

_____

_____

_____

_____

What kinds of reminders do you need to keep doing them?

_____

_____

_____

_____

_____

_____

Have you made feeling good a priority in your day?

_____

_____

_____

_____

_____

Having Fun

What do you do to have fun?

_____
_____
_____
_____
_____
_____
_____
_____
_____

Are those things fun for your Inner Self too?

_____
_____
_____
_____
_____
_____
_____
_____

What kinds of fun did you have as a child?

_____

_____

_____

_____

_____

_____

_____

_____

_____

_____

"Make space in your life for the things that matter, for family and friends, love and generosity, fun and joy. Without this, you will burn out in mid-career and wonder where your life went." —JONATHAN SACKS

Can you create moments of that kind of fun now?

How can you make having fun a regular part of your days?

Reflections

What surprised you about yourself these past two weeks?

_____

_____

_____

_____

_____

Did you learn something new?

_____

_____

_____

_____

_____

Can you put your new awareness into action?

_____

_____

_____

_____

_____

Satisfaction

What do you do that gives you satisfaction in your life?

_____
_____
_____
_____
_____
_____
_____
_____

Are you satisfied in your work?

_____
_____
_____
_____
_____
_____
_____
_____

Are you satisfied with yourself?

Are you satisfied with your relationships?

"Success is finding satisfaction in giving a little more than you take."

–CHRISTOPHER REEVE

How can you create more satisfaction in your life?

_____

_____

_____

_____

_____

_____

_____

_____

_____

_____

_____

_____

Gratitude for Doing the Work

How would you like to show gratitude to yourself for doing the work in this book?

_____

_____

_____

_____

_____

_____

What is your favorite way to show gratitude?

_____

_____

_____

_____

_____

_____

_____

How can you do that?

_____

_____

_____

_____

_____

_____

_____

_____

Can you express gratitude to God, your guardian angel, or whatever higher power you trust?

_____

_____

_____

_____

_____

_____

_____

_____

_____

_____

Is there anyone in your life you'd like to express gratitude to?
What would you say?

"Develop an attitude of gratitude,
and give thanks for everything that
happens to you, knowing that every step
forward is a step toward achieving
something bigger and better than your
current situation." —BRIAN TRACY

Reflections

What surprised you about yourself these past two weeks?

_____
_____
_____
_____
_____

Did you learn something new?

_____
_____
_____
_____
_____

Can you put your new awareness into action?

_____
_____
_____
_____
_____

Who Are You Now?

Read over the past prompts and your answers in this book.
How has your thinking changed?

_____

_____

_____

_____

_____

_____

_____

What are you doing or thinking differently about?

_____

_____

_____

_____

_____

_____

How has your relationship with yourself changed?

"The greatest discovery of all time is that a person can change his future by merely changing his attitude." —OPRAH WINFREY

How do you feel?

_____

_____

_____

_____

_____

_____

_____

Who are you becoming with the new changes?

_____

_____

_____

_____

_____

_____

_____

_____

_____

_____

A Job Well Done

Congratulations! You've come to the end of all fifty-two weeks, and hopefully, you are proud of yourself. Remember, you can go back over any of the weeks that seemed most helpful to you or that you wanted to do more. Good mental health is worth working on for a lifetime.

Have you accomplished what you were hoping to accomplish with this book?

_____

_____

_____

_____

_____

_____

_____

_____

_____

_____

_____

_____

_____

_____

What would you like to keep working on?

How do you want to celebrate your accomplishments in the fifty-two weeks?

> *"To be yourself in a world that is constantly trying to make you something else is the greatest accomplishment."*
>
> —RALPH WALDO EMERSON

Using what you learned in Week 24, design a celebration to acknowledge what you learned and achieved.

_____
_____
_____
_____
_____
_____

How would you like to give thanks?

_____
_____
_____
_____
_____
_____

Final Reflections

What surprised you about yourself this past year?

_____

_____

_____

_____

_____

Have you put your new awareness into action?

_____

_____

_____

_____

What positive changes do you anticipate this new awareness
will make in your mental health and in your life?

_____

_____

_____

_____

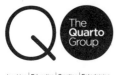

Inspiring | Educating | Creating | Entertaining

Brimming with creative inspiration, how-to projects, and useful information to enrich your everyday life, quarto.com is a favorite destination for those pursuing their interests and passions.

This edition published in 2023 by Chartwell Books,
an imprint of The Quarto Group
142 West 36th Street, 4th Floor
New York, NY 10018 USA
T (212) 779-4972 F (212) 779-6058
www.Quarto.com

10 9 8 7 6 5 4 3 2 1

Chartwell titles are also available at discount for retail, wholesale, promotional, and bulk purchase. For details, contact the Special Sales Manager by email at specialsales@quarto.com or by mail at The Quarto Group, Attn: Special Sales Manager, 100 Cummings Center Suite 265D, Beverly, MA 01915, USA.

ISBN: 978-0-7858-4189-0

Publisher: Wendy Friedman
Editorial Director: Betina Cochran
Senior Design Manager: Michael Caputo
Editor: Jennifer Kushnier
Designer: Sue Boylan

Printed in China

This book provides general information. It should not be relied upon as recommending or promoting any specific diagnosis or method of treatment for a particular condition. It is not intended as a substitute for medical advice or for direct diagnosis and treatment of a medical or psychological condition by a qualified physician or therapist. Readers who have questions about a particular condition, possible treatments for that condition, or possible reactions from the condition or its treatment should consult a physician, therapist, or other qualified healthcare professional.